This is Going to Help:

HOW TO SURVIVE AS A JUNIOR DOCTOR

Dr Moushmi Biswas

Dr Anna Scholz

DEDICATIONS

To Dr TK Biswas, much loved Anaesthetist and Dad
To LM, my rock, Dr LL an amazing teacher and JS, a
wise friend

CONTENTS

FOREWORD

It was after I read Adam Kay's '*This is going to hurt: Secret Diaries of a Junior Doctor*', that I felt compelled to write this. I loved the book. It was funny. It was poignant.

It was also very disturbing.

Why did such a bright, talented and dedicated doctor leave the NHS at the beginning of his career? What kind of example has he set for the rest of our fledgling doctors who might be tempted to jump ship?

The mere mortals amongst us who aren't blessed with other skills. Like being able to write comedy for television for instance.

There are many of us who have trained in the pre-European working time directive era. We have worked the kind of hours Adam describes in his book and faced similar challenges. Yet we went on to have successful careers. We've also had families, pursued creative interests, won awards (not me), done research, travelled the globe and even gone on 'Bake off' (not me).

Unfortunately, not everybody managed those things.

Many of these folks got completely sucked into the vortex of 'being a doctor in the NHS'. Many of them blundered through year by year, without a plan or direction. Some became so involved in hospital life that they forgot to live their own.

And you only ever get one.

It is mentioned in self-help books that there are two parts to climbing a mountain, the journey up, and admiring the view. As a junior doctor you are on that steep, rocky climb. You will feel sick, frustrated and overwhelmed. You will have doubts about ever reaching the top. But this is the most exhilarating bit. And you are at your youthful best!

This book contains snippets of real experiences, personal stories and some savvy ideas on how to live well and work effectively. We are not experts and you may not agree with everything!

As your senior colleague, I'm grateful to be able to share them with you and hopefully, ease your journey through this phase of your career.

Dr Moushmi Biswas, Consultant Physician

FOREWORD

The stereotypical view is that doctors work all the time. But we don't. We get time off and a good amount of leave. Not always when our friends are free, but we do. We work with kind and intelligent people. We have job security and job satisfaction.

But we can also reach a point where we become deeply unhappy and feel like quitting.

I love my job. I love life and I have great friends. But there have been times when I've cried while driving to work, felt physically incapable of getting out of bed to catch a flight and I've even vomited. Why? Because I was so darn tired. And I was partly responsible. I am greedy. I want to do and have it all.

Exhaustion can make us feel overwhelmed. A lot of it is to do with our shifts. But often, it's our own selves. Doctors are high achievers. We have high standards. Sometimes when we want to give, there are things beyond our control, like lack of beds and staff sickness. When patient care gets affected, it affects us. We try to maintain our life and commitments outside of work too, then everything just crashes.

After going at 110%, mini-crashing, recovering, going 110% and mini-crashing, I finally listened to my mother, when she said, "Sometimes Dr Busy should timetable in doing nothing."Just nothing.

So sometimes, I would sit at home and do nothing. It was surprising how many spontaneous mini-adventures would pop up!

Now, I try and factor in "buffer zones" of chill time before and after a heavy on call block. And I've realised that I don't have to be perfect at everything, in work or outside of it.

I just need to be good enough in that moment, for that moment.

Being a medic is a vocation, but YOU are more than just medicine. Hopefully, this book will help bring some balance into your life. What we've written is based on experience and observation. We don't have all the answers, but where we've discussed problems, we've also talked about how to try and tackle them.

In that way, this book is different to other junior doctor books. Also, because it concentrates on YOU.

The YOU outside of work.

Dr Anna Scholz, Specialist Registrar in Diabetes and Endocrinology

CHAPTER 1

TICKING THE RIGHT BOXES

Real conversation.

MB: "Congratulations X, I am so happy to hear you have a consultant job in a teaching hospital now. I can't believe you used to be my SHO!"

X: "I still haven't filled those boxes you talked about."

MB: "Did you at least learn to drive?"

X: "Er… No."

MB: "*%&£"

I used to do this exercise with my juniors when I was a medical registrar, before they started a six-month rotation. I knew all along who would drift and who would flourish.

These are not drunken New Year's resolutions. These are real aspects of your one and only life. No one can fill these boxes for you. And if you don't fill them, it is nobody else's fault.

Exercise: Sit down quietly for ten minutes and ask yourself how you would like to fill each of these boxes in the next six months of your life. If you are not sure, leave the box blank.

Health	Career	Academic	Family	Social	Adventure	Hobbies	Financial

Now let's break these down

Health

Firstly, you should be looking after yourself, drinking enough water, moving your body and eating healthily. It is very tempting to comfort eat when you are stressed and running around. I got to a size sixteen doing that and then my health goal became 'getting to a size ten'. At least set a realistic goal, like, 'I won't eat rubbish from the vending machine'. And do some type of 'movement' activity. Not using the lifts, which are frequently out of order anyway, counts more than unused gym membership, (see finances section). And there are plenty of 5-30 minute on-line workouts, where you can do anything from Aerobics to Zumba in the comfort of your own home, before work!

AS: Rotas can make joining a regular club or class difficult. Difficult but not impossible. Group activities can be fun and allow you to 'plug in' with new people. Even a twenty minute walk a few times a week counts as ticking the health box. Use your smart phone to track your steps!

Career Progression /Academic

This is your NHS ePortfolio and how you should be filling it in as you go along. We will come to how you can time plan for this in another chapter.

Family

You must try your best to make time. Even when you are on nights. Meet for breakfast! If your folks live overseas, aim to visit. Schedule in face-time calls. If you have kids, try to have some uninterrupted time out with them. Please. It is easy to forget that many non-medics 'out there' face job stress, work shifts and juggle families, some with chronic illnesses too. We are all busy, so that does not cut it as an excuse.

AS: I'm really close to my Mum and it's usually a relaxing time popping round for a cup of tea, but we've worked out that if I meet up with her on a Friday evening at the end of a busy week on call, I am tired and grouchy. It's completely different after an evening to myself. I'm much nicer and way more fun! It's striking that balance between caring for your loved ones and looking after yourself.

Social

You've got an audit to complete, you are preparing for PACES / OSCE and a week of nights is coming up. How do you make time for social activities? Buddy up! Find at least one person and say, "Right we'll see some cases together and work on this audit and then we'll go for a meal. And during the meal…we will not talk about exams. Or the audit.

People complain that they lose touch with friends during the junior doctor years. Who are your really close friends? How will you make time for them?

A trick I still use is to meet 'in the middle' for a coffee at a McDonalds before work starts. For privacy, you can drink it in one of your cars. Nowadays video chatting is a good tool also.

AS: Trying to co-ordinate meetups between a group of docs can be tough with everyone on different schedules. My group of friends would take it in turns hosting 'Bake Off' or the 'Apprentice'. If one of us couldn't make it one week, then we would join the next. It was a great way of getting fed and chilling out!

But trying to fit everyone else in can be hard. A date with your sofa now and again is not so bad either. If you are constantly having a date night alone, ask yourself why? Are you slipping into a downer? Are you exhausted? Has anxiety about meeting people/self-image crept in?

Adventure

Human beings have always been in search of it. At the very least, go visit some place different that you haven't been to. You do not have to go far. Even going for a 3-mile hike in a wood that you've never explored counts.

AS: My 'one day crash course in crime writing' was great. It took me out of my comfort zone gently and showed me that I was capable of other things outside of medicine.

Hobbies

My Dad's was reading the newspaper everyday from cover to cover. He was an Anaesthetist. He squeezed it in, between cases and of course, during. As a time-starved junior doctor, you probably won't have time to paint sellable water colours. But you can find something simple like listening to a podcast or reading the paper. Use the same thing across boxes, (eg: hiking in the woods with friends counts as being healthy, sociable and as a hobby).

AS: Being an F1 was all consuming. The main topic of conversation always seemed to be medicine. As an F2 I went to Barcelona and signed up to some Spanish guitar lessons. I loved it and I'm still having weekly lessons on Skype. My teacher is really flexible around my shifts and not having to leave the house is one less stress! There are a lot of things you can learn on Skype these days. Having a different headspace keeps me fresh.

Financial

Many doctors are bad at this. Get a financial advisor. I mean it. If you haven't got one, ring one and make an appointment now. They can tell you about ISAs, income protection and mortgages etc. Two things I will suggest. Before you start a new rotation, go through the direct debits in your bank account and delete the ones you don't need (eg: unused gym membership). Also, frittering away your week's earnings on expensive coffee and treats is really daft. Forty quid a week is easy to fork out. Now do the sums: F1+ F2 + CT1.

AS:Mobile banking apps, like Monzo can track your spending. It's so easy to get into the habit of spending what you earn. As your salary goes up, your spending goes up. I learned to transfer some of my money into a savings account as soon as I got a pay increase, so I didn't get used to splurging with the extra income. I do allow myself nice holidays though and a cleaner twice a month!

Membership fees and exams will eat into your disposable income, but you can claim such costs against tax. You only have four years though and I missed the boat! The link below can help.

https://www.bma.org.uk/advice/employment/tax/junior-doctors-tax-guidance

Another thing

If you are in a team of junior doctors, why not try to help the people in your team achieve their goals alongside yours? Talk about important goals with each other beforehand. Passing PACES. Taking time off to visit a sick relative. Getting married.

AS: I always found that it made sense to join in with other members of the team for things like 'audits' and 'quality improvement projects.' It's sociable and you get more done in less time.

Suggestion

When starting a new rotation, Registrars drag your team together! Each member in the team reads out one sentence stating their major objectives in the six-month period, (work-related and outside of work). One sentence only please. Preferably without any narcissistic twaddle.

AS: Doing this over a team dinner outside the hospital is a bonding bonus!

Exercise for you. How do you intend to fill these boxes next week?

Health	Career	Academic	Family	Social	Adventure	Hobbies	Financial

CHAPTER 2

YOUR MENTAL HEALTH

Entrepreneur and founder of Mindvalley, Vishen Lakhiani once asked each member of his audience to turn to the person sitting next to them, smell them and describe the smell. Thankfully, people smelt of exotic berry shampoos, Lynx deodorant, and Chanel perfume. He was trying to convey an important fact. We are all prepared to spend time, money and effort on toiletries, but how much are we prepared to invest in taking care of our own minds?

Doctors are particularly bad at this. We take on everyone else's problems. We have challenging jobs. We witness death and suffering day in, day out and regularly experience failure. And for junior doctors there are other stressors which may affect mental health, such as disrupted sleep, exam stress and repeated moves.

Drink or drug problems

Dr G: "It started off as a social activity and a form of stress relief. We all did it in those days. But of all the things I regret about drinking… the people I've hurt, the driving bans…what I regret most of all is the time I wasted sitting in pubs, night after night, talking complete bollocks. Time I will never get back…"

Doctors are at high risk of drug and alcohol misuse. There are a number of reasons for this, which include: 'accepted' medical school behaviour, job stress and ease of access. Fear of consequences may lead to delayed disclosure and this has far reaching implications.

You may have a drinking problem if you:

Feel guilty or ashamed about your drinking

Lie to others or hide your drinking habits

Need to drink to relax or feel better

Forget what you did while you were drinking

Regularly drink more than you intended

Or, when you clerk patients with an alcohol related admission and realise you would probably answer 'yes' to most of the questions you asked them before writing up their Pabrinex and Diazepam.

Where do you go?

Drinkchat and Drinkline are free confidential help-lines for discussion about one's own or someone else's drinking. You should also see your GP who can refer you on. Each Deanery also has a Professional Support Unit (PSU) to help trainees who are struggling with problems that prevent them from achieving their training goals. You will have access to quick referrals and a team who will understand the unique stressors which can affect doctors. We will discuss the PSU in more detail below.

Anxiety and Depression

Sometimes you may be unsure as to whether anxiety and low mood are a normal part of your training years, or whether the problem is more serious.

Normal anxiety - situation driven and short lived

At a cardiac arrest

Before exams

Before an important Interview

Abnormal anxiety - seemingly for no reason, disproportionate to situation, difficult to control

Before coming to work

When out with friends at a social event

Fear of putting in a venflon, taking blood or something you have done hundreds of times

Get help

There is nothing to be ashamed of. Many of us will face severe anxiety in our lives and require treatment. Even the greatest surgeons can 'lose their bottle.' If you are unsure as to whether you have 'normal' anxiety or an abnormal level of anxiety, you must talk it through with your GP or Occupational Health Physician. Once again, do not let things escalate. Unfortunately accessing counselling services through a GP can take several months, so this is where the Professional Support Unit can be invaluable.

Anxiety from making mistakes

Sadly, this kind of thing has previously led to doctors taking their own lives. We have all made mistakes and so will you. Fortunately, in most cases there will be no major harm done. Very, very, very occasionally there will be. It is recommended that you join a defence union, see the link below. It will cost you, but once you do so, there is someone at the end of a phone who can talk you through the situation in confidence. There are other support services offered, like counselling. Also, you will feel a little peace of mind knowing that you have legal protection.

https://www.gmc-uk.org/registration-and-licensing/managing-your-registration/
information-for-doctors-on-the-register/
insurance-indemnity-and-medico-legal-support

The Professional Support Unit

Dr O: "After having a bad time with exams and in work, I became anxious and depressed. I self-referred to the PSU after finding that NHS options were very limited. I was seen by their lead Mrs L, who referred me straight onto a Psychologist who specialised in treating doctors. The PSU funded a full course of CBT for me and they have also given me help with exam skills. You can email them directly and they find the right person to assist you. I would certainly recommend this service and wouldn't hesitate to use them again."

Professional Support Units (or PSUs) are designed to help support doctors during training. The PSU can work with a trainee and link in with the Deanery and Occupational Health if needed. In some Deaneries, around 10% of trainees are receiving support from the PSU at any one time.

PSUs provide help for doctors experiencing a wide range of issues including ill-health, personal problems, acute crises or organisational concerns which are impacting on wellbeing and training.

The PSU can also assist you if you are struggling meeting the ARCP requirements, or with getting feedback on assessments. And if you are an international medical graduate who has not previously worked in the NHS, you can even access 'cultural coaching.'

You can access the PSU by checking out your Deanery's website.

AS: I only heard about the PSU recently after talking with friends who have had anxiety or bereavements which began to affect them in and out of work. They spoke highly of the counselling they received from counsellors who had worked with other doctors, so they actually understood what "F2" or ARCP meant. Some people have even chosen to continue their counselling sessions privately on a long-term basis, as it enables them to manage the stressful or upsetting aspects of a job they love.

BMA Counselling and Doctor Advisory Service

If you are not happy at work, it will impact on your home life. If you are not happy at home, it will impact on your work life.

Did you know that as a member of the BMA, you have 24/7 access to a telephone counselling service? They are there for you if you have issues at work, concerns about your family, or children, or if you are experiencing a crisis in your relationship.

Their phone number is 0330 123 1245.

Positivity and Gratitude

In an organisation like the NHS where services are greatly stretched, it is easy to forget about any good work which is done. Yet each day babies are born, life-saving operations are performed, people with acute illnesses are cured and people with chronic conditions are surviving longer and longer.

Instead we habitually moan about how bad things are. I've heard people refer to situations as 'like a war zone'. Casualty may be busy, but we have to remind ourselves it is not a war zone.

Maintaining a sense of humour, staying upbeat, positive and expressing gratitude can really help shift your own mindset and that of your team. Why do the self-help people talk about gratitude so much? Because when you are grateful, you cannot be angry or fearful. And suddenly, your perspective changes.

Now I am not saying that you won't have days which are overwhelming, frustrating and upsetting. Nor am I saying that you should try to be funny in the middle of an emergency or use self-help jargon on a distressed relative. I am showing you some tools which will help you get through the difficult times.

Guided meditation and mindfulness have been shown to reduce stress, improve well-being and aid sleep. These techniques are several thousand years old and not harmful. Increasingly, they are being used by athletes and performers to improve clarity and mental focus. There are apps you can use and plenty of free content on You Tube.

In the past, many people in the medical establishment were dismissive about all this 'voodoo psychology' stuff. They came up with phrases like 'you've got to get on with it' and 'see one, do one teach one'. And their philosophies were simply handed down to the next lot of suckers.

But if these techniques can help 21-year-old soldiers in real war zones, run through searing deserts wearing 60-kilogram backpacks, or by an actor with stage fright make his Broadway debut, then why can't they help junior doctors?

Suggested Meditation apps and videos:

The six-phase guided meditation by Vishen Lakhiani

A blend of relaxation, personal growth and creative visualisation

Duration: 13-20 minutes

Stages: 1. connection (reminds you of how you are directly connected to every life form)

2. gratitude (expressing thanks for 5-10 things in your life, big or small)

3. forgiveness (bringing to mind conflict and apologising)

4. visualising your perfect future (how you would like your life to look 3 years from now)

5. setting a daily intention (all the things you would like to achieve in the day)

6. blessing (calling on any higher power you believe in, or your own inner strength)

Headspace

A popular guided meditation app with graphics, run by a former Buddhist monk

Duration: ten-minute sessions with reminders during the day

Motivational videos

There are many worldclass motivational speakers who have trained everyone from Hollywood A-listers to US Navy SEALS. Their books, audiobooks and You Tube videos may be a valuable resource to help you with things like:

- Priming yourself mentally for exams and interviews
- Restoring your self confidence
- Making life decisions
- Stress and depression

AS: A book I found really helpful was 'Manage your Mind: The mental fitness guide', by Gillian Butler and Tony Hope, a Psychologist and Psychiatrist respectively. It was really practical and it provided excellent tips on how to look after your mind.

Examples of Motivational Videos

Marissa Peer: transformational psychologist who uses hypnosis and other techniques.

Topics: self-esteem, helping you train your mind to achieve success, losing weight

This lady's methods have helped thousands of Hollywood A listers. And she is rather unique because she uses 'Rapid Transformational Techniques', which work very quickly to 're-programme' your mind in contrast to the traditional 'lay on the couch once a week for years' model of therapy.

Tony Robbins: entrepreneur, philanthropist and life coach

Topics: how to become disciplined, achieving wealth, changing the way you feel, achieving success

One Navy SEAL had Tony Robbins piped through his headphones while he was in the helicopter on his way to capture Bin Laden.

Ted x Talks

These are short, but powerful talks on subjects related to technology, entertainment and design. There are also useful presentations related to self-improvement and great little videos with catchy titles, such as, 'On being wrong' and 'How to stop screwing yourself', as well as the more serious topics such as 'The art of the interview'.

CHAPTER 3

PLANNING THE WEEK AHEAD

PLANNING YOUR WEEK: a Consultant's perspective

The successful person makes use of his time successfully. At induction you should have received a weekly timetable outlining the ward rounds, clinics and theatre sessions for your team. I suggest you use an electronic diary or draw up your own timetable to include the tasks which you have to complete every week. I am not saying that you stick to it religiously, but you should have a rough idea. Remember the boxes in chapter 1 and try to incorporate other aspects of your life into the timetable.

Golden tips: If you get the difficult or unpleasant stuff out of the way first, you start off on a 'winner' and the rest of the day runs a lot smoother. It is particularly useful to get things like 'exercise' or 'exam revision' out of the way before you come to work, or even your ePortfolio.

These are the areas that are most likely to suffer after a busy day at work. Sometimes it might make more sense to get to the hospital early to grab a parking spot then find a quiet place to do some revision. If you are in a hospital with a gym or a pool and you wish to exercise, then coming in early to complete a couple of sessions before work is also a good idea.

I have constructed a timetable below as an outline. Obviously in surgical jobs you will need to start earlier and if you really want to stay on top of things, go to bed earlier too!

Time	Monday	Tuesday	Wednesday	Thursday	Friday	Saturday	Sunday
6-9 am	Park Run	Revise	Park Run	Revise	Revise	Park Run	Sleep in
9am	Ward round (stairs)	Consultant ward round (lifts!)	On call until 9pm	Ward round (stairs)	On call Until 9pm	MOT car Haircut	On line banking
	Team Lunch	**Team Lunch**	**Own Lunch**	**Free Lunch**	**Coffee Treat**	**Own Lunch**	**Lunch Out**
2pm	Ward jobs 2 DOPS (Directly Observed Procedural Skills)	Ward jobs QIP (quality improvement Project)		Teaching Attend Clinic		Football with mates	Food shop
6pm	Revise	See Mum	1 ACAT (acute care assessment tool)	Chill Session		Night out	Plan next week Revise

What is expected of a junior doctor in a surgical job?

Mr W: "At this stage I would prefer it if they used their stethoscope properly. Only then will I let them go near a scalpel."

- Surgeons like to know that you can take care of their patients before and after an operation.

- They like you to know about the patient they are about to operate on.

- They also like you to know about the operation they are about to do.

- Some of them are also interested in writing research papers

Three things that really irritate my surgical colleagues:

- Juniors showing up to operations without reading up about the operation or the patient

- Being called about sick patients who have not been assessed and had the basic ABC started

- Aspiring surgeons who only want to operate and who are uninterested in pre/post op care

An efficient surgical trainee will:

- Get the weekly timetable from the consultant

- Get a print out the week's operating lists

- Schedule in time to read about the operations beforehand (even on your phone)

- Know about the patient undergoing the operation (especially their previous medical and surgical history and scars)

- Ensure that sick patients on the ward have been seen before striding into theatre

- Communicate with relatives politely

What if you are an F1 who is not interested in a surgical career?

Your time in a surgical job will be invaluable if you use it to:

- Get experience in dealing with medical problems single-handedly (remember you can always ask for help from the medical team / seniors!)

- Practise cannulation, arterial punctures, nasogastric tube insertion etc

- Expand your CV with a small project

GETTING HELP WITH TIME CONSUMING ACTIVITIES

Many time starved junior doctors often ignore a really valuable resource: the established, well settled folks who work in the hospital. I mean the senior doctors, nurses and secretaries. Most people would know of a trusty car mechanic, decorator, hairdresser, dog-walker or plumber. It can sometimes be overwhelming if you run into a problem when you have just moved to an area, so just ask. Some might give discounts for NHS staff as well.

Also, you could save money by walking into the hairdresser around the corner straight after work and you'll avoid the rush hour. Or you could take your car into a garage nearby, which offers lifts to local employees. Otherwise these jobs can eat into your weekend (as in the table above).

How to fit in revising for post graduate exams. (Just when you thought it was all over...)

You have probably developed a routine at school and university of going to classes in the day and coming back home and revising. Word of caution: after a busy day at work, you may find yourself too drained. And if you are unprepared, you won't pass. Taking re-sits really drags out your training years. What about sleeping early and starting your revision at

0600 am? Make use of the library for private study at lunchtime if you can. Remember most trusts find it difficult to accommodate more than a day or two of private study leave.

AS: I found that breaking it all down into smaller chunks made it easier to start and achieve. Also, when I left the house earlier, before the traffic started, I could get some proper studying done before work started and that way I could enjoy my evening.

PLANNING YOUR WEEK: A junior doctor's perspective

"No man is an island." John Donne (1572-1631)

You are working as part of a team. Some days there will be plenty of bodies on the ward, other days there will be few. Before starting the week, find out how many team-members will be around. Then get your system in place. Now, on your own:

- make a list of urgent and semi-urgent tasks (See "master list" in Chapter 4)

- make a list of non-urgent tasks that can be done when there are more people around, or if the ward is calm

Remember:

- If you are short staffed, try and complete the urgent tasks and semi-urgent tasks.

- If there are lots of people around, you can tackle the non-urgent tasks as well.

How?

When the ward is calm, and there are lots of bodies around, try to make sure that the jobs are distributed so that someone can do the routine ward work and someone else can carry on with the non-urgent tasks that lie waiting. Send a team-member off to a quiet place, where they can bat through some discharge summaries or phone relatives. Find someone else who can go down to clinic, or work on the team audit.

Getting to clinic

This can be difficult but it is a crucial part of training. It can be easy to get caught up on the ward and miss clinics. Then weeks pass by. Unwell patients take priority, but people often avoid clinics because they feel guilty about leaving their colleagues on the ward.

Plan out clinic attendance at the start of the week. You can see which days are better staffed and factor in who went to clinic last week. Even if the team is busy, one hour away from the ward is manageable.

If it's a morning clinic, you can bypass the ward and go straight there. This way you cannot be easily diverted. You have to be reachable in case there is a real disaster or if your colleague on the ward needs help.

If it is just you on the ward, this can be really difficult. First talk to the charge nurse, the Registrars and to your Consultant. If there are no acutely unwell patients, you might still be able to pop down for an hour first thing in the morning. I've held bleeps for my SHOs just so that they could get to clinic.

To get the best out of clinic in a short time:

Find out about the three most common conditions seen in that clinic. Read up on them beforehand. Patient.co.uk or Up to Date can provide a quick overview, even as you walk down the corridor!

Clinics are a great way of getting to know your Consultant, getting your assessments done and they give you an insight into what a specialty is really like.

For example, as a junior doctor you may be completely put off by a career in specialties like Oncology or Diabetes and Endocrinology, because you have only seen these patients on the ward. And they all seemed to have had insurmountable problems. By attending clinics, you will get a taste of the 'success stories' and phenomenal preventative work that gets done in these specialities, which may completely change your outlook.

CHAPTER 4

PLANNING THE DAY AHEAD

PLANNING YOUR DAY: tips from a Consultant

"One of the habits of very successful people is that they do what they don't like to do first."

Marissa Peer,
Transformational Psychologist.

The start time of your ward round will vary depending on which rotation you are in and generally tends to be earlier in surgical specialties and anaesthetics.

A handover

In many wards an initial board round is undertaken to identify which patients are sick and which patients are going home. It is usually required that one or more doctors, a charge nurse or two and a bed manager attend. These meetings should not last more than 15 minutes, but I have seen them being used as a forum to discuss any topic from how to get Ed Sheeran tickets to bizarre patient antics. I suggest you ask yourself one question before you start the handover:

"Do I want to get home today?"

The daily ward round for a medical team (Consultant led or not):

A ward round of up to 25-30 inpatients should not take more than 3 hours. An efficient way to get around is to see patients in this order.

1. Sick patients (wherever they are)

2. Those people going home (Bed managers like it the other way around!)

3. Outliers

4. Patients in your base ward (starting with the cubicles)

Why is this the most effective way?

- The sick patients can be dealt with swiftly, investigations arranged, outreach teams notified and ceilings of care determined. It gets people home quicker and creates beds.

- If you begin by seeing every patient on your base ward, it is difficult to avoid being interrupted as you go around and this will delay you getting to the outliers.

- Medical outliers are patients who belong in a medical ward, but who have been 'outlied' to a non-medical ward, such as ENT, due to a bed crisis (the crisis seems to be happening daily). Surgical outliers are less common. Nurses looking after outliers might be out of their comfort zone and need your guidance. Such patients may complain about their care. Now does it make sense as to why they should not be seen at the end when you are flagging!

Lunch time

Many hospitals will have lunch time teaching sessions at least a couple of times a week and you should try and attend, particularly if Drug Reps or the Postgraduate department are offering you a free meal. At least twice a week I would recommend having a 'social lunch' with your team. Be conscious of time though.

The afternoon

This time is usually reserved for talking to relatives, procedures, clinics and chasing blood tests. Try and allocate a specific amount of time to try and finish things eg:10 minutes to write blood forms for the next day. Half an hour for discharge summaries.

But a junior doctor's life is unpredictable and patients do become acutely unwell and new ones can enter the realm at any moment.

Many Consultants won't mind if you take it in turns to leave a little earlier. That is, if your work is finished, you have not left very sick patients unattended and there is someone to cover you. This should be discussed with your seniors.

Time wasting and gossip

"Did you hear about so and so?"

I have known doctors and other staff who stay back late into the evening on a daily basis. Interestingly, they don't get seem to get much more done than the rest of us.

Between coffees, cigarette breaks and extended lunches, a lot of time can get wasted. And one big time-waster is gossip. Before you indulge, please remember the following:

1. What you hear may be untrue and can be harmful.

2. Even if it is true, today's news becomes tomorrow's fish and chip paper.

In order to achieve work-life balance as a junior doctor, try to remain

- mindful of those boxes in chapter 1 and time conscious.

AS: Gossip can be negative, but asking about nurses' kids and holidays is positive. Showing a bit of interest in people makes the work place more cohesive and dispels the views that some docs can be standoffish. If you aren't into social chatter, then bringing the odd treat in for staff or offering to help sit a patient up shows that you are part of a team. I try to be friendly with the nurses and I try and help them. In return, if I'm rushed off my feet they help me.

PLANNING YOUR DAY: A junior doctor's perspective

Boardround/morning handover (Shout!)

Quick, structured succinct. 10-15 minutes. Everyone understands what the priorities are, you can flag up the medical concerns and avoid Chinese whispers.

Take turns leading the board round. It's a useful experience even as an F1.

The way to keep it moving along is to just shout out the name of the next patient after the major issues affecting the previous patient have been discussed. Sometimes I think there is room for a little bit of chitter-chatter! Sometimes things that happen are funny or sweet! Just remember the longer handover takes, the longer your day.

So, keep shouting! Politely, of course.

Daily ward round (it's all about the patient list!)

Designate the list keeper and if it's you, get in a few minutes early. Yes, getting in early is not 'regulation', but if you start the day organised, you will get home on time. I would definitely arrive earlier on Mondays, as there will be a lot of new patients. Rule: whoever comes in earlier, gets to leave earlier sometime that week.

Identify the new patients and if you are in early, you can sweet talk the phlebotomists into taking their bloods. Getting in early is good for patient care and you will know about your patients beforehand, and get 'brownie points' in front of your bosses. Check for outliers.

Assess what the day is looking like. If there are no dramas handed over, then set an aim to have a rewarding 'tea or coffee' if the ward round is completed by a certain time. This really focuses the team and makes them more efficient. Discharge summaries and management plans will get finished a lot quicker!

During the coffee break, you can put together the 'master list', which I'll tell you about soon. A shared 'cuppa' is really good for team bonding too. A bonded team is a happier team. And happier teams mean happier patients.

Early discharges

If there are plenty of doctors on the ward, then send a couple of them out during handover to get on top of the day's discharge paperwork and take-home medications, so Pharmacy can get it all ready.

This means patients get home earlier. It keeps Bed managers happy. More importantly it means Mr Smith who's been sitting on a chair in A and E all night can get a bed.

It also means that new patients arrive on your ward during working hours. This way you can become familiar with the patients and do their blood forms ready for the next day.

If discharges are delayed

The later people go home, the later the new patients come to your ward. You encounter them the next working day. As you don't know them, you appear clueless on the Consultant ward round. And worst of all, as you haven't had a chance to give the phlebotomists their blood forms, you'll end up having to do the bloods. This really delays things and drags out the whole day.

So, which is better? Coming in early, knowing the patients, getting their forms and investigations done and getting home quicker? Or having to rush round cluelessly, having to do everything yourself and playing catch up?

Before lunch: the most important time of the day

- Get the ward round done before lunch. If you are flagging, have a 5-minute break for a snack or rehydration. Then keep going. It's much better for patients and it makes your afternoon smoother.

- Get the Radiology requests in. An early request can mean the scan gets done in the afternoon, rather than next week. I don't know why but this seems to be a universal rule in Radiology!

- Before leaving for lunch, check that the ward patients are 'ok' and ask the ward to make a list of non-urgent jobs which you can tackle after lunch.

- If there is a very sick patient who is acutely unwell, it often only needs one doc to stay back and sort them out, so the rest of you can go to lunch.

Lunch

Have it. Have it. Have it. Preferably off the ward for a change of scenery. It's also nicer to have it together, then you can concentrate on the 'master list' (coming up soon!). Add on a bit of time for a cup of tea too. Bringing your own lunch will save you money. This way if a disaster strikes, you will not starve, or worse, gorge on chocolates and then face the accompanying sugar crash.

Afternoon

- Check blood results before 3 pm, so that you can identify and treat any abnormalities quickly.

It's not fair if you only check blood results just before 5 pm, then hand over the management to the on-call team. Like for instance, the low potassium, or the sudden rise in creatinine.

- Once the urgent jobs are completed, arrange to speak to families. Aim to do this before 3 pm and definitely not too close to leaving time. Not only because you want to get home, but because any issue they flag up won't be dealt with until the next day. If you are busy, get an idea of their main concerns, document them and arrange a more convenient time to speak. Or better still, take their phone number and offer to call them.

- A controversial idea is to ask someone to bleep you 15 minutes into a conversation with a patient's family. Otherwise, things can go around in circles and it's hard to know how to end things without appearing rude. The bleep serves as a time reminder. If the conversation is productive and you feel it is helpful for the patient's care, then you can always carry on.

Handing over to the on-call team

It is their job to work that evening. YOU are allowed to hand things over and GO HOME! But within reason. If there is a delay in lab processing and a blood result is not back, that is reasonable. If there is a sick patient who requires another review, that is fine as well.

If you are handing over things that should have been done in the day, you need to think why. Either you need to speed up, or prioritise. Or is it a staffing problem? Speak to a senior about it and they can give you tips. The first year can be overwhelming and simple tasks will take longer.

Not leaving on time – every day

There will be times when a patient suddenly goes 'off' just before five or when your ward jobs get delayed because you had to attend a teaching session and a clinic. In extreme circumstances you will have to stay back. But if you fall into the trap of getting in super early and leaving late every single day, you will burn out. Your life outside medicine will suffer and you may have to go off sick. Nobody wins.

When I did a job in which there were gaps in the on-call rota and permanent staff shortages, I acknowledged the problem and asked for help.

I canvassed the rest of my team's views, including my Consultants' and I sent an informal email to the deputy Clinical director. The statements I made were calm and logical and most importantly, non-blaming. A meeting was set up, the situation discussed and as a result we were given a locum SHO for the rest of the rotation. Wow! What a difference!

Daily staffing issues and how to handle them

- Let your Consultant know and they can escalate it

- Discuss the option of cutting clinics/ theatre time (management really hate this!)

- Ask if it is possible for outliers to be given to teams with greater staffing numbers

- No blaming, shaming or complaining. Simply record and present the facts. How many patients are there? How many doctors? How much sick leave was taken? How many clinics are trainees missing? How might this affect the upcoming GMC training survey?

- Find a quiet, calm space away from the turmoil and document this information in a polite email so that your concerns are on record.

- Please remember that angry emails shot off in the heat of the moment can make things worse. Other people are stressed too.

- If you are really angry and upset, leave the ward and go to the toilet. Find someone to talk to, like your Mum or a senior colleague. Rants, tears and histrionics leave a lasting impression. Surgeons seem to get away with it, but unfortunately not junior doctors.

The Master List

Ward jobs generally include making Radiology requests, putting in specialty referrals or asking for phone advice. You will also be writing discharge summaries and prescribing take home medications. Sometimes there might be a few miscellaneous chores like having to call a relative to get a collateral history or to arrange a time to meet.

By the time you have jotted down all the jobs on your computer-generated patient list, you may be left with a mess of scribbles. On busy teams, with large numbers of patients or when you frequently have to cross cover with another team, making a 'master list' of jobs can really streamline your afternoon. Do it over your 'reward coffee', or at lunch.

I came up with the idea when there were three of us juniors looking after a busy 30 bedded ward. Initially, so we could get things done, one of us would run off with Radiology requests or one might be called to take urgent bloods. Because the whole team weren't on the ward round, it was difficult to know what had been done and what needed doing. Someone might have been down in Radiology chasing a CT scan, but then an urgent ultrasound generated from the ward round would be missed. Someone would be waiting on the phone for Microbiology advice about one patient and later someone else would be doing the same for two different patients.

Making a master list ensured that there was only one trip to the Radiology department and one phone call to Microbiology about three patients. Less running back and forth. Less hanging on the phone. Less time wasted! Now share out the tasks. Anything outstanding can stay on the list for tomorrow.

Example of a Master list

<u>Referrals</u>

□ Micro: Beds A1, C3 & D1

□ Chase Vascular Bed D4

<u>Miscellaneous</u>

□ Collateral History for C2

<u>Take Homes/Discharges</u>

□ D4

□ B5 (for tomorrow)

<u>Radiology</u>

☐ CT Abdo bed A2

■ CXR B6

<u>Bloods</u>

□ Which phlebotomist couldn't do

□ or abnormal results which need actioning

Weekend day ward cover

This gets easier as you become more senior, you do things more quickly and become more confident at prioritising.

Handy hints:

1. make sure you carry food and water. You can always get water from the kitchen, but I usually carry a protein bar or two in case I get stuck with a sick patient

2. check bloods as early as possible so you can bleed the patients the phlebotomists have missed and identify any abnormalities quickly. It's not good to discover a serious problem at 7 pm, 9 hours after the blood was taken.

3. Get a batch of empty sticky labels, find somewhere quiet, like the mess, and write out the name, ward number and any abnormal results. This way, as you go around the wards the sticker can be put in the patient's file and the abnormalities actioned.

4. When handing over to the weekend team, do not simply write 'check U and E' on patient X. Please write why you need the result to be checked and what to do afterwards eg:

"Check U and E and CRP on Patient X with pneumonia. If CRP / U and E improving, no action needed. If worsening, please review Patient X.

Managing expectations and answering your bleeps

Nurses do not know where you are or what you are doing. For all they know you could be watching football in the mess. Nurses usually have 6-10 patients each and you are responsible for many more. They spend all day with the same patients. So, if a patient is angry or agitated it's much harder on them. Imagine being on the receiving end the whole time! Also, if they tell you that a patient is deteriorating, believe them.

If you can't come right away, take a few seconds to explain why. Ask what the patient's observations are and not just the NEWS score (National Early Warning score which indicates how sick a patient is). If you are given the NEWS score, ask what it normally is. This helps you to triage. If it is not an emergency, explain that you will be there in X number of hours, but ask them to bleep you if the patient deteriorates or if you haven't arrived by X time. Write this down on your list. If they bleep back in twenty minutes, you will realise that this patient has deteriorated.

State at the very beginning of your shift, that you are happy to be bleeped by the nurses if the problem is urgent. Explain that bloods or cannulas can mostly wait (unless it's a blood transfusion or antibiotics for sepsis). Tell them you will get to them faster if you are only bleeped about urgent things. For non-urgent tasks, ask them to prepare a list, explain that you will be doing a tour of the wards and tell them roughly when you will reach their ward.

This gentle education will definitely cut down the number of bleeps you will receive over a weekend.

Asking for help

Don't be afraid to ask, but remember weekend staff are thin on the ground and busy. At first, find out the ceiling of care. You should not be fast bleeping the Registrar about deteriorating blood gases in a patient with end stage COPD, on maximal treatment, when the Respiratory team have already stated that the patient is not for HDU, ITU or Non- Invasive Ventilation. Try to triage.

Simple non-urgent questions: batch them together and touch base with seniors regularly so you can discuss them eg: choice of antibiotics or can this patient be discharged or can he eat and drink.

Urgent questions: Assess and treat the patient initially yourself. Giving fluid boluses, placing them in an appropriate position and Oxygen therapy can rapidly make a patient better without senior review. Do this first, as well as requesting bloods, gases, ECG and CXR if required. Have notes, investigations, drug charts and bed charts to hand before making the phone call, as you will be asked lots of questions. Basically, the person you are speaking to is also triaging. Be succinct. For example:

"I am an F2 calling for an urgent review of patient X, with hospital acquired pneumonia. He is for full active treatment and his BP is low and HR fast despite a fluid bolus."

Really sick deteriorating patient: If someone is so sick that you don't even have time to do the basic ABC and initial management, then it is a peri-arrest situation and you can call 2222. Use this resource wisely. I've seen people call 2222 because it gets an Anaesthetist over to help with a venflon.

Not good.

The NHS ePortfolio: A junior doctor's perspective

The NHS ePortfolio and Turas often feel like a box ticking exercise and can be a real source of frustration. It's also hard to set aside time when it's busy. But it's important, as it provides a record of what you have achieved and proof that you have completed your required competencies.

It definitely isn't worth the panic and despair the week before ARCP, when you realise that you have loads to sign off! Suck it up. Do little chunks of it over the year. Slot in a little time for it every couple of weeks in your weekly time-table. Then it's only a minor annoyance, and it allows you to focus on the areas in which you need more experience.

What I've learned from my supervisors is that people don't engage very well with it. So, if you do a little bit here and there, you already look good.

Handy hints on managing this monster

- Record clinics and send assessments on your ePortfolio or log book before you leave work.

- Sign into your ePortfolio when your assessor is right there. No sending tickets or reminders then.

- Find a carrot. Meet friends for coffee with your lap-tops and all of you do 15 minutes of ePortfolio stuff before hanging out. My carrot was reality TV. I allowed myself to watch low-concentration, trash TV while filling in my 'reflections'. That way, my ePortfolio was quick and painless.

The NHS ePortfolio: A Consultant's perspective

Prof K: "I had written down NOT ONE thing. All my work over the years. Where was it? I began to panic. I couldn't sleep. Revalidation suddenly took up eight whole weeks of my life."

I do think the ePortfolio is a lot of red tape, but guess what? It doesn't go away. As a Consultant or GP, you will be asked to fill in appraisal forms on-line. If you haven't got the right evidence, it will affect your revalidation, and ultimately, your right to practise.

Each year, you will have to submit a tax-return and gather documentation for that. Also, if you do private practice then you will have to keep records of patients, invoices, income and what not.

In fact, you will probably be recording, submitting and box-ticking for most of your adult life.

If you can acquire the discipline of keeping records and doing things 'bit by bit' now, it will help you a lot in future, so you won't be rushing around in blind panic before a tax deadline or appraisal date.

Building your CV: A junior doctor's advice

Audits: Group together. This way you can get your name on more than one audit or include a larger number of patients which looks better on your CV because it provides more meaningful results. I also find I am more likely to get a project finished this way.

Short listing scoring systems for future specialty: These change year to year, but look at what they are interested in. You will have to complete a quality improvement project, but you will score more points if you actually present it at a conference. If you have scored enough points, then you don't necessarily have to do another one. Presenting at your team's weekly teaching session may earn you a good number of points and possibly even more than an intercalated degree would.

Building your CV: A Consultant's advice

Written publications tend to carry a lot of weight in a CV. It was not until I had my first Case Report published that I figured out why. Writing a paper, even a Case Report, is a painfully slow process which requires attention to detail and focus. It showcases your writing skills, as well as your dedication and perseverance, because it can get rejected so many times! The higher the 'impact factor' of the journal the better, but generally anything in print attracts attention.

I personally believe that a single, properly conducted audit of a large number of patients is far better than three poor quality audits with only ten-fifteen patients in each. A large audit can even double up as a retrospective study, and eventually become a written publication.

Oral Presentations and Poster Presentations at Regional or International Conferences also embellish a CV nicely. We discuss other ways to build up your CV in Chapter 9.

A word of caution

People in other professions often boast about 'lying on their CV'. There have been desperate trainees who have lied about audits and publications. If the Training Committee suspects falsification, they will contact the GMC. These guys take any dishonest behaviour pretty seriously, as we are expected to act with honesty and integrity as doctors. It would be a shame if you worked hard and passed all your exams, but were then declared unfit to practise because you lied about having a paper accepted.

CHAPTER 5

GETTING THROUGH WINTER AND NIGHTSHIFTS

Are you winter ready?

Imagine you wake up with a temperature of 38 degrees, a dry cough and a pounding headache. You have run out of paracetamol and milk. It is 1 degree outside and the last thing you want to do is drive to the supermarket, but you have no choice.

STOP! REWIND! That would never happen if you were winter ready! I would recommend that you tick off this checklist when the clocks go back at the end of October, particularly those of you who have not experienced a British winter. I wish I'd done this as a junior doctor. It would have saved me a lot of misery!

And I'm not being facetious when I mention the team lunches and dinners. This is a particularly busy time of the year, particularly for paediatric and medical teams. Respiratory illnesses are abundant, patients are scattered far and wide. Staff sickness is also common and you may be forced to cross cover and do marathon ward rounds across the entire hospital. Any form of morale boosting is most welcome!

Winter checklist	Tick off
Winter coat and gloves	
Winter shoes	
Winter tyres /tyre check	
Anti-freeze	
Blanket in car	
Long life milk	
Ready meals/ frozen food	
Store cupboard stuff (pot noodle / tins)	
Torches / spare light bulbs	
5 boxes of Lemsip in different flavours	
Night Nurse – cold remedy	
Flu vaccination	
Team Festive lunches	
Team Festive dinners	

PREPARING FOR A WEEK OF NIGHTS:
a junior doctor's perspective

Food

- Buy it at the start of the week. Try not to shop on your way home from a night shift. I have left the supermarket with 2 for 1 DVDs, a giant stuffed pug dog (it was on sale) and a strange assortment of food.

- 'Easy to prepare' is the key. Batch cook or buy healthy ready meals and accompany them with salads. If you don't have food at home you will be tempted to stop off at McDonalds or Greggs on your way home, which is guaranteed to make you overweight and spotty.

- Eat enough before going to sleep. It's very upsetting to wake up hungry at 3 pm.

- Get some 'good to go' food ready for your night shift. Bananas, protein bars and Tupperware filled with cereal are all good for this. If you make batches of sandwiches and freeze them, they can defrost quickly. Warning! This only really works for ham, cheese and peanut butter sandwiches. But it also works for buttered hot cross buns too. Yum!

Entertainment

I need something to help me unwind pre and post night shift. Either a light-hearted movie, or the latest box-set. You can meet people for an early dinner before nights. But keep it simple and don't commit. You may wish to see how you feel at the time.

Sleeping

Before nights: get a good night's sleep the night before. I've tried going to bed really late to get myself into 'night mode', but I still ended up waking at the normal time. So, this just made me more tired before starting a shift. Different people have different body clocks though. You have to find what works for you.

During nights: I like to have the morning to myself, watch TV and nibble until midday then go to sleep for several hours. This way I get a couple of hours in the evening before work. Others go to bed straight away. Once again, you will discover what is best for you.

Tips to help you sleep during the day

- An eye mask

- Black out blinds/ curtains

- White noise. A door banging or your house-mate coming in can wake you up. Get a track with 'sudden sounds', such as thunder over the ocean. This way you will block out bangs and other sudden sounds.

- A boring podcast or audio book on low volume can help if you are struggling. It's stressful to be lying there thinking *"I'm still awake. I'm still awake"*, but if you have to concentrate on someone speaking, you'll slowly drift off.

- Friends have tried anti-histamines, but they can make you groggy. Never drink alcohol. It messes up your REM sleep and it can become a dangerous crutch.

On your night shift:

Have a break. You are meant to have half an hour every four hours of working. If you are hungry, thirsty and sleep-deprived, you won't think straight. Look at the guidance given by the Royal College of Physicians. Using part of your break to have 15 minutes of shut eye, even while sitting in a chair will help you function better. Just put your phone alarm on and make sure you are not sitting on your bleep. Registrars make sure the team gets their breaks.

Getting home:

Most people just want to get home. But I know people who have crashed their cars from microsleeps. They were okay, but other doctors have died. It's why we pay more for car insurance.

Having a cup of coffee a couple of hours before going home can help (remember caffeine has a 5-7 hour half-life). Sometimes a 15-20 min nap before driving off is the safest option.

The BMA rules state that you need a minimum of 11 hours between shifts. So, if your hospital insists that you must stay for the entire post-take ward round, point this out. I won't stay past 10 am anymore, as by that time, I am barely able to speak.

CHAPTER 6

MAKING CAREER CHOICES

Dr R: "I hated nights and on-calls so I left hospital medicine to become a GP. I had no idea I would spend ten hours a day sat at a desk with no one to talk to but the receptionist. I ballooned in weight from sitting all day. I felt lonely and isolated. I was gutted when I realised my mistake. The nights would have ended once I'd finished my training! I joined a Hospital Rheumatology clinic once a week and spent one day in A and E. This re-established my social network. Eventually I figured out that I could make more money working just three 'out of hours shifts' a week in General Practice. So that's what I do now."

MB: "£$&*!*$£!"

Dr L: "I couldn't pass my Membership exams, so I was unable to get into specialty training. I became an Associate

Specialist instead. Eventually I got my Consultant job through Article 14. It took ten years, but I stuck with it and I'm so glad I did."

Once upon a time, after you completed your training, a job in medicine was forever. These days there are many options and we're far more flexible. Being stuck in a job or career you don't like can feel like falling down a mineshaft. Please remember there is always a way out. Always!

There are two ways you might go about getting out. Sometimes it makes sense to stick with something until you have a qualification. It will help build your CV when applying for new jobs. Sometimes it's better to quit outright. You have to decide what is right for you.

I have met GPs who re-trained and became extremely successful Radiologists. I have met Physician trainees who have gone onto become truly great GPs.

There are also people who have a career portfolio rather than a single job. For example, they might be a GP for part of the week, an appraiser for other GPs for one day and a sports doctor the rest of the time.

Helping you choose

The British Medical Association website contains excellent career advice for medical students and doctors. It includes video presentations on different specialties and they have also developed a psychometric test that helps people choose a specialty based on their personality type. I have jotted down a list of questions and considerations, but would strongly recommend that you visit their website.

Questions to ask yourself

1. Do you like working in a team?(Diabetes)

2. Do you like working with your hands? (Surgery)

3. Do you believe in a holistic approach to patients? (Care of the Elderly)

4. Are you prepared to work nights and on-calls for the next thirty years? (O and G, Anaesthetics)

5. Are you prepared to stand up for long hours at a time and operate? (Neurosurgery)

6. Do you like new technology? (Intensive care, Cardiothoracic)

7. Do you like working with children? (GP/ Paediatrics)

8. Do you prefer slow paced work (Palliative care, Elderly care) or

9. the adrenaline rush (Intensive care)

10. Would you prefer an exclusively 9-5 job? (Rehab medicine)

11. Do you like medicine and surgery? (Ophthalmology)

Other considerations

1. Would you like to make a lot of money? (Orthopaedics, but not Rehab medicine)

2. Are you prepared to perform the same task over and over?(many cystoscopies in a row)

3. Do you prefer working in a setting where there is no direct patient contact?(Pathology)

4. Would you prefer dealing with simple solvable problems(Dermatology) or are you fascinated by complex problems (Neurology, Psychiatry)

5. Would you prefer working in a private setting all of the time? (Dermatology but not Renal)

Tweaking your career

Your medical career can be divided into a few stages. Firstly, there will be your junior doctor training years. Then, after completing your course requirements and passing exit exams you will receive certification enabling you to practise as a GP or Specialist. Subsequently there will be an early career stage, mid-career stage, a period of sabbatical leave if you choose and the chance to 'downsize' pre- retirement. Some people prefer to work a little after retirement too.

Working in the NHS can offer you the kind of flexibility that many careers simply cannot provide and you can tweak your job as you go along. The BMA and various Royal College websites provide detailed information on the subjects discussed below, but here is a guide.

Working as a Consultant

Your working day will be split into 'sessions' and each session lasts 3-4 hours. Depending on the terms and conditions of the Consultant contract in the part of the UK you work, there will be an expectation that you perform several sessions of 'direct clinical contact' in one week.

These sessions include things like operating theatre time, ward rounds, outpatient clinics, reviewing investigations, pre-operative visits and on-calls. You will also be given time for Supporting Professional activities 'SPAs', like preparing teaching sessions, undertaking research and for clinical management. You might even be allowed to complete some of these sessions at home.

After fulfilling the Trust's service needs it will be up to you to negotiate the rest of your job plan and SPAs. And each year you will have an appraisal and review of your job plan. If a particular part of your job is not working out, you might let a colleague 'take that session' and do something else.

Working as a GP

You may wish to work as a 'salaried GP' with a fixed salary, contracted duties and hours. Or you may want to become a 'GP partner' where you take on more responsibility for running the practice and earn more, with a share of the profits. Or you can work as a Locum GP, in different places. You may start off one way and change paths.

Handy Hints

- If you like a particular field you can be a GP with a special interest, such as Diabetes, Dermatology or Neurology. You can do specialist courses without full specialty training.

- Some careers may begin with a rigorous initial training period, as in Paediatrics or Obstetrics and Gynaecology. You can later become a Community Gynaecologist or Community Paediatrician, in a relaxed clinical setting, without on calls.

HIGH INTENSITY CAREERS

Obstetrician's son: "My father was always being called. Women can go into labour at any time and he had lots of private patients. He would leave during my birthday parties, football matches and school assemblies, then go off in the middle of the night. It would upset me. At eight my mother moved me to a Private school and both of us stayed in an apartment nearby. We visited Dad on weekends and it was easier to spend time with him that way. But even so, he'd get called out."

There are certain jobs in the medical field which are 24-7. Obstetrics, Neonatology, Critical Care, Transplant surgery and Cardiothoracic surgery to name a few. Before you think of going into such a field consider the implications on your lifestyle. Also, if you are really passionate about a particular specialty, ask yourself:

1. What appeals to you about this job as a medical student/junior doctor?

2. What will the job be like in specialty training? Can you see yourself doing it as an ST?

3. What will the job be like as a Consultant? Can you see yourself doing it several years from now?

Some careers appear glamorous as a medical student, but the day to day reality is rather different. Ask a Specialty trainee in one of these fields what life is like for them. It may be difficult for you to speak to Consultants directly, but you can certainly find out from Specialty trainees what life is like for their Consultants. Please try not to base choices on the 'Superhero' image, it's unrealistic.

And remember if you really enjoy working in a particular field and choose to follow your heart, you will have to find your **own form of work life balance**. Go back to the boxes in chapter 1. Your boxes will not look the same as everybody else's, but every life is unique.

There are other professions, such as politics and the armed forces which are arguably associated with even greater disruption to people's lives.

p.s. The Obstetrician's son mentioned above has become a very successful dentist and enjoys a very happy relationship with this father, who at the time of writing has refused the option of retirement.

If in doubt try it out!

AS: Remember, people like to be martyrs, so they tell you that their job is the hardest. I tried to fight against becoming a medical Registrar. People told me it was one of the hardest jobs in the hospital and that no-body wanted to do it. I had all my exams and a good CV, but I decided against committing to specialty training straight away as I wanted a period of time to 'try out' being a medical Registrar. I discovered that I really enjoyed it. That time won't count towards my official training, but it has made specialty training much easier! And I had a year without the ePortfolio!

CHAPTER 7

THE RING-FENCED YEARS

Mr W: 'Surgeons cannot have their training handed down to them on a plate. We came in on weekends to follow up the patients we had operated on. We asked to be paged when we were not on call to do cases. We practised and practised. That's how we became good at our job.'

Dr R: "When my Dad got sick, I couldn't fly over to visit him. It was the last month of my fellowship at the Massachusetts General Hospital. Every minute counted. I spoke to him twice a day instead."

Dr F: "Once I started my PhD, I had to finish it. It sapped five years of my life. I missed many, many weekends with my kids. In the end, I didn't really need the degree. It made no difference to my job title, or my pay. I got three letters next to my name, but my youngest hardly knows me. I wish I'd thought about it more before enrolling."

In order to achieve something, you will have to make sacrifices. Beyoncé didn't become Beyoncé overnight. She has been at it since she was four years old, made sacrifices and overcome her fair share of hurdles. Nothing comes from nothing.

If you want to be really good at something or if you want a special qualification, you might be required to 'ring fence' a certain amount of time in your life where one particular goal will be the predominant focus. For this you will have to be a little selfish. And your work-life balance will appear more 'work-work'.

Remember the longer you continue in this 'zone', it is likely to affect other aspects of your life. There are some things that you can make up for in future. But there are some things which you can never make up for, such as not being around for your children. Or not having children.

You can still come in on a weekend for an hour or two to follow up the patients on whom you have operated. You might want to do it early, before a day out with the kids. It won't always be possible though and there will be things that you will miss. If you have partners, you must communicate!

Before you embark on a major undertaking, such as accepting a job with a lot of travelling, doing an MD, or travelling abroad for a fellowship, go back to the first chapter on 'TICKING THE RIGHT BOXES'.

What will you have to forgo in order to achieve your goals? How long are you prepared to forgo these things? Importantly, will it be worth it?

Exercise: Ask yourself these questions and jot down brief answers.

What is it that I would like to undertake?

_____

_____

What do I hope to achieve by this?

_____

_____

How will it impact my family?

_____

_____

What can I do to make it easier for my family?

_____

_____

How will it impact my partner?

_____

_____

What can I do to help my partner?

_____

_____

How might it affect my finances?

_____

_____

What steps can I take to protect my finances?

_____

_____

How might it affect my social life and hobbies?

_____

_____

What can I do to maintain some form of social life?My hobbies?

_____

_____

How might it affect my health?

_____

_____

What can I do to protect my health?

_____

_____

CHAPTER 8

DATING AND RELATIONSHIPS

Dr P: "I knew I could never manage a relationship when I was in training, between the on calls, the moves and the travelling. So, I decided to put it off. When I became a GP, I chose to work two days a week and the rest of the time I devoted to on-line dating. I know it sounds like a lot, but you need time to get your hair done, exercise and look your best, before even going out. It took me three years, but then I met S and we have two lovely children now. A girl and a boy."

Dr A: "I am here on a two-year fellowship. My boyfriend lives overseas. It is hard, but we have concentrated on making it work. We face-time each other through the day, have NETFLIX nights and schedule our holidays together every 2-3 months."

Dr S: "When I work late shifts on the weekends my husband cooks me a meal and brings it in. We try and eat together."

Many of you have been lucky enough to meet your significant other in University. So, by this time your relationship should have a solid foundation. Dare I say, you are a 'smug married' and the major decisions are 'wood or laminate?' Or 2.4 children or 3.2?

But for the junior doctor in a newly established relationship, or on the dating scene, the situation is more fragile. You may find yourself on a perilous journey through random hook-ups and forgettable flings. And unwittingly, as a source of entertainment for smug marrieds.

Things to think about

Before you are ready to 'give' to someone else… are 'you' okay?

- do you have a job and a place to live?

- a rough idea of where you will be heading in the next 6-12 months?

- a close set of friends / family around / hobbies and interests

We are back to the boxes in chapter 1. A relationship is one component of a balanced life. All the other things are your safety net in case things go wrong. Even so, breakups suck. Be realistic though, if you have just accepted a surgical training job in Edinburgh and the person you are seeing is staying on in Hull, then you are skating on thin ice.

Dating

AS: Planning ahead seems a bit commitment-heavy, romance lite, especially at the start of a relationship, and particularly if you are seeing a non-medic. However, shifts limit spontaneity and your social calendar can be quickly filled. It's frustrating to miss out on times where you could have seen each other, but you didn't, because you were playing it cool. Suddenly it's three weeks later and all momentum has gone. I haven't quite cracked this one. My married friends are disciples of synced Google calendars for work and play, which allows them to maximise time with friends or alone time as well as time together.

If you are just about to start a busy rotation with a lot of travelling, then it may not be the best time to look for a serious relationship. There may be an easier stint sometime during your training or, have you considered taking a year or two out for research? Your timetable will not be as packed and this way you can really throw yourself full throttle into internet dating.

Also, you may meet a whole new bunch of people in a University, or through the 'research community'.

The Doctor-muggle (non-medic) combination

Doctoring has its unique aspects, but despite how it's portrayed in TV hospital dramas, at the end of the day it's a job. It has particular demands and responsibilities and it can be inflexible at times, but it should not be seen as being more important or special than your other half's job. Again, communication is the key here.

The Doctor-Doctor combination

Despite all the swiping right and left which goes on these days, 40% of female medics still marry another medic. I always felt that it made sense. You mixed in the same social circles. You shared the same morals and ethics, liked helping people and could both earn a decent living. In addition, you understand each other's job pressures. If either of you is called out unexpectedly midway through your Michelin star restaurant meal, you get it. And if someone is shaken up by something particularly traumatic that happened that day, you will listen quietly, without mentioning the leaking bathroom tap.

There are downsides, for which you may want to consider casting your net wider. In reality, there is almost always a downside to just about anything. It doesn't have to be a deal breaker. Sometimes just knowing what you are signing up for helps.

The perpetual work and patient centric conversations

If both of you enjoy it, then it's fine. But it can be tiresome if one of you (like me) doesn't. You will just have to learn to set limits and boundaries. Like, not while stood in front of a Monet at the Musée d'Orsay (true story, with whispered commentary). Not even over a cappuccino in the Musée d'Orsay.

Shared skillset, but not the right ones

You both want a dream home. Neither of you have the time, energy or knowledge to go about creating it. You are reliant on various tradesmen, each of whom has a unique and highly individualised concept of time. Neither of you can supervise them because you're at work. Your dream home becomes a nightmare. For years.

I know of an Ophthalmologist who took evening courses in plumbing and electrics to overcome this problem. By the time he retired, his house looked great!

Childcare

If you don't have willing and able family members around, this can turn out to be a very expensive juggling act. There is before school care, after school care, at least thirteen weeks of school holidays plus several inset days. In the NHS, our 6 weeks' annual leave entitlement is more generous than in many professions, but it is difficult to take more than 2 weeks off at a time.

Remember someone in the teaching or academic profession might earn significantly less, but may be able to give a child added parental time, which is priceless.

AS: It used to be the mother who would go part-time. Increasingly parents are sharing this. If you are both trainee doctors, rather than one going 60% and almost doubling the training time, it can make sense for both parents to go 80%. This way both parents can get added time towards their training and two extra days of childcare. If you want to find out more, the links below are useful.

https://www.gov.uk/childcare-calculator
http://www.medicalwomensfederation.org.
uk/advice-support/childcare-advice

CHAPTER 9

LONELINESS AS A JUNIOR DOCTOR

"The world is suffering from an epidemic of loneliness."

-Vivek Murthy Former US Surgeon General.

This is not a problem confined to older people. Coming to a new country, starting a new job in an unfamiliar place or unsociable working hours can result in loneliness and isolation. And because it's embarrassing to admit and hard to recognise, it can be a difficult condition to treat.

Staying back at work can be a very convenient way to both hide and tackle loneliness. The hospital is a warm, well lit-place, filled with people and activity.

You can be sitting in a ward, working on an audit, or writing up a case. The nurses ask you to join them on their tea break. Three months down the line you are caught in a vicious cycle. You are lonely because you cannot meet people outside the hospital and you cannot meet people outside the hospital because you are always in the hospital.

And it is through this process, that you risk becoming institutionalised. I have worked for a Consultant, on a seven-figure salary, who always ended up sleeping in 'Recovery' and not at her beachside apartment.

Everyone is different and there are some who may prefer to live this way. But if you wish to expand your horizons and experience a broader life, then you will have to leave your comfort zone to beat loneliness.

And while going to the gym and running on a treadmill wearing earphones counts as exercise, it is not a method for treating loneliness. So, come on everybody and get out there!

Group Activities

Most places in Britain will have leisure centres and or community centres that run many activities, mostly for an hour or two. They are often subsidised and sometimes there is no membership fee. If you are on a budget then you can join the activities in which you only pay each time you turn up. That way if you miss some days due to your on-call rota, you won't be penalised.

Examples of community centre activities include:

Chess clubs, Yoga, Zumba, Allotment gardening (learning to grow fruit and vegetables)

Book clubs (usually monthly though)

Then there are other groups such as football teams, cycling and cricket teams and also the famous 'Ramblers', a walking charity which provides guided group walks through the British countryside.

There also are a number of 'Meetup Groups' which pop up through social media, for people with a common interest. The meetings usually take place in a café or pub. I've been invited to Book clubs, Chess clubs and Political discussions through social media.

Volunteering

There are many wonderful organisations in the UK which offer you the opportunity to volunteer. This is a great way to fill your time, meet people, serve the community and expand your CV. You can look for volunteering opportunities in line with your hobbies and interests. For example, you could work with a wildlife charity if you like animals. Or you can choose something which is more in keeping with a future career, for example, becoming an 'event volunteer' or 'speaker volunteer' for Diabetes UK.

My experience as a volunteer for Cardiff Institute for the Blind (MB)

I had to get a criminal record-check and undergo a four-hour training session on a weekday, during which I learned about the organisation, the daily challenges affecting a blind person, how to help them and how to guide someone while they walk. You got to try on different spectacles which enabled you to 'see' the world through the eyes of someone with tunnel vision, hemianopia, cataracts and macular degeneration. Just that little action itself had a profound effect.

There were activities for 'full time volunteers' in the centre such as teaching computer skills or gardening. The activity which best fit in with my working hours was the 'befriending' service, so I joined that.

Once a week I would visit an elderly lady for an hour or so, read her mail or take her out to lunch. She would always pay her way. But do you know what really made a difference? It was not my sparkling company!

The carers who did her food shopping were on foot, so they could only buy her stuff from the tiny local shop. If I was visiting Marks and Spencer or Waitrose, I offered to pick her up a few bits and bring them over when I saw her and she'd give me the money. She said it was life changing!

Volunteering was an extremely rewarding experience, and not onerous at all. If I was away or busy, I didn't do it. I gave it up after three years when I began going through the adoption process, but one day I hope to pick it up again.

The Loneliest Time of the Year

If you have family, friends, young children and pets, Christmas in the UK can be an amazing experience. But if you are a junior doctor, separated from your loved ones, it can be absolutely awful. And it's worse than Valentine's day for singles, because it's dark and gloomy and it drags on for several days, during which your mates might be away.

If you can't be with your friends and family, because they live overseas etc, I strongly suggest you offer to work and allow someone else to have the time off, so they can be with theirs. This way you will be busy, included in the ward festivities and be able to tag on two days of annual leave when you want to go away. When the fares are a lot cheaper.

Suggestion

Before you start a six-month job, plan out the working arrangements over the Christmas period. If your family live overseas, you could offer to work over Christmas and schedule a visit home earlier in the year. Like during Eid or Puja/Diwali if it's more appropriate for you.

If you do have to stay back over Christmas, ask other people if you can join them, or use that time to study or finish a work project. If you are bored or lonely, those of you from outside the UK may not know about the world-famous post-Christmas sales. You start by queuing around the shops in the early hours of the morning with other excited bargain hunters. The Selfridges and Next sales are quite an experience! But these days, most people just go on-line.

CHAPTER 10

HAVING CHILDREN—OR NOT

Dr N: *"We knew we wanted children, so we had them early. My husband was working, so I had the first child mid-way through medical school and the second in core training, with the benefit of paid maternity leave. When I went back to work, my eldest entered school and the youngest went to nursery. We could not have afforded to have both in full time nursery."*

Dr I: *"I wanted to wait until I had a stable job, a house in the golden triangle*and no on calls. I had all that as a Consultant, but the baby wasn't happening. We tried IVF, unsuccessfully. It was soul destroying. Then we went through the adoption process and we got our beautiful baby boy of three months old. Six months later, I was pregnant!"*

During my training years, it was difficult and almost frowned upon to take maternity leave. Thankfully, the NHS has been at the forefront of making positive changes to help junior doctors if they choose to become parents. The 'ideal' time to have children is a very controversial and emotive subject.

For each 'time zone', meaning the 20s, 30s and 40s, there are different issues which may crop up, but they can be dealt with. Everyone's journey towards parenthood is different and there is no right or wrong way or time. When kids come along, you'll just end up working around them. Below we give you some food for thought, and that is really all it is.

the distance between your place of work, kid's school and home, ideally like an equilateral triangle. The shorter the sides the better for work-life balance.

In your 20s

Fertility is optimal at this point and you've got your whole life ahead of you! But trying to fit in training, night shifts and taking care of a baby can be extremely stressful. A career break might be an option, but that may affect your finances. Also, some of my friends who had their children 'early', complained that their forties were just a 'sequence of losses', with menopause, ill parents and kids fleeing the nest.

In your 30s

People might be more settled in this age group and the bulk of training / exams may have over. After the mid- thirties, some people may face a rollercoaster ride trying to become pregnant. Egg freezing is currently expensive and success rates are low.

In your 40s

You are likely to need assisted conception and the success rates are higher with donor eggs, resulting in a 'non-biological' child. This also applies to the adoption route, which you may be required to take. If you don't consider this to be a deal breaker then it's not a problem.

AS: The best piece of fertility advice I've heard was from a kick-ass female Obstetrics Consultant with four kids who taught me at med school. She always said "there is no convenient time to have a baby". She had seen many female registrars in her fertility clinics, each one upset that they may have missed out on having kids because they were so focussed on their careers. And all them had waited for the right time that never came.

If it is important to you, then try not to put it off. You've got decades of your career ahead! And if you're not sure, or don't want them, you could just go with the flow!

Planning maternity leave and returning to work

You should initially read the document entitled 'General Maternity Guidance for rotational Junior Doctors in training'. This gives you information about when to notify employers, when you are able to take maternity leave (from around 11 weeks before the baby is due) and the two different payments (occupational maternity pay and statutory maternity pay) and who can claim. There is no information on how you should plan things over the course of your pregnancy. Although each person's pregnancy and career path are individual, below I've outlined a rough guide. Men should contact their staffing department about planning parental leave as well.

Example of a timeline during pregnancy

- 8-2 weeks register with midwife

- 12-15 weeks inform team and employer (earlier if you are unwell)

- 20 weeks obtain MAT B1 certificate (to access maternity leave and pay)

- 32 weeks, come off on call rota (if earlier, then need GP/Occupational health review)

- 32- 36 weeks, sign off e-portfolio, finish clinic letters, discharge summaries, paperwork

- 35- 36 weeks, start maternity leave. You will also accrue annual leave in this year.

Example of a timeline before returning to work

- 4-6 weeks before starting, get timetable and rota, leave contact details, sort childcare & hols

- 2 weeks before starting, touch base with person currently in post, find out what's expected

- 1 week before returning to work configure all NHS passwords, dry-clean clothes

- Day before starting work, hoover and clean car and get petrol (from Mums Net!)

AS: Choosing when to start maternity leave is a balance between having that final bit of 'me time', preparing the nest and spending time with your new baby. The link below contains some very useful advice on maternity leave and pay.

http://www.medicalwomensfederation.org.uk/advice-support/maternity-advice

Adoption leave

One person out of the couple is entitled to 52 weeks of adoption leave. The other may take parental leave. You will have to obtain a 'matching certificate' fromyour adoption agency and provide it for your employer in order to access occupational adoption pay and statutory adoption pay. Your social worker can help you plan your timeline before going off, but it is generally only a matter of a few weeks rather than months.

A career break

Dr P: "I had three children fairly close together, so I decided to take 5 years off. It was very hard to get back in. I had to do exams, retrain and revalidate with the GMC. If I had known about all the hassle, I would have taken 3 years off and not 5."

Increasingly career breaks are being taken by men and women for a variety of reasons other than for having children. If you wish to take a break, consult your postgraduate department or relevant Royal College beforehand. You will need to know if your ability to revalidate could be affected and how to manage appraisals. It is also worthwhile checking in periodically to make sure that the rules about returning to work have not changed.

A child free life

There is still a societal assumption that every man, woman or couple wants a child and this is simply not the case. Comedian Sara Millican does an excellent stand-up routine about it. If you choose to be child free, beware of having to take on extra work to cover someone else's maternity leave or because someone is coming off the call rota. Make sure you speak to medical staffing about remuneration. Half terms and school holidays can be difficult too, as you may feel like the only person around. But you will make up for it by taking your own restful holidays, at a quarter of the price.

AS: Offering to babysit your friends' kids can be really fun, earns you brownie points and you get to hand them back before sleep time! It can also be a 'taster session' for what to expect if you are undecided about having kids.

Pets

A pet is for life, not just for Christmas. It can be nice to come home to a warm furry body, but pets need a lot of attention. Food, water, worm and flea treatment, Vet visits, exercise and company are just the basics for dogs. I would only suggest that you get a dog during your junior doctor years if you are able to care for it jointly with your partner, or if you have family around to share the care. Even doggy day care and walkers will not be enough to see you through shift work and trips away. Cats need less care, but they can get lonely too. And remember many rental properties will not allow pets of any kind. It's also worth noting that just paying for food, Vet bills and pet insurance may cost you a couple of thousand pounds a year.

AS: Offering to walk a friend's dog when you can, or pet sitting for them if they go away is a great way to enjoy time with dogs and cats, without the full commitment. This is a useful link if you are interested.

https://www.borrowmydoggy.com

Coming back to work after you have had children

Congratulations on becoming a parent! Your life has changed and your priorities have changed. But don't expect everyone to 'get it'. Most of them will not have a clue, and will not 'get it' until they have kids one day, if they ever do.

Things you might want to think about:

- If you are considering coming back less than full time, you will have to give your employer at least three months' notice, but the longer you can give the better

- By now you are an expert at 'the thirty second blast shower' and the 'leap out of bed without a lie in'… are there other ways you can save time?

Time saving tips

- Buy non-iron clothes.

- Plan meals for the week, then do on-line shopping for the ingredients all in one go.

- Run errands at lunch time if you can (post office, dry cleaning).

- Get workwear, baby clothes and tomorrow's food ready the night before.

- Use time saving apps such as to do lists and the Tesco Groceries App.

These time saving tips seem just as good for people without kids as well!

A useful link

http://www.medicalwomensfederation.org.uk/ advice-support/return-to-work-advice

Emergency leave

You may have to take time off if your baby/child is ill and thankfully in most cases it might only be a day or two, but your colleagues will probably find it difficult. The shorter the notice, the more the disruption and tempers may fly. When my son had to have emergency surgery on his hand, the clerical staff weren't exactly compassionate. But I understood that it was because they were tasked with ringing patients (many of whom were on their way in), to cancel them. If you have to take leave and other staff are not that gracious, don't take it personally. When you come back to work, try and make it up in some way eg:

-   By holding a bleep for the person who covered you and allowing them to leave early

-   Offering to take them on a PACES teaching session, or helping them with an audit

-   Doing some ward jobs and discharge summaries for them

-   A jar of coffee and a box of tea for the clerical staff and of course, biscuits

Special occasions

If you want to attend your child's Christmas concert, don't expect everyone to jump through hoops for you.

I remember asking my Registrar to hold the fort when I attended a concert and I cross covered her so she could attend her child's concert. It was only for two hours or so, but if you can find someone in the same situation, you could mutually benefit.

CHAPTER 11

WORKING SMARTER

Work-life balance is not just about living well. It's also about working well. This section is designed to help you work more efficiently and effectively as a junior doctor in the NHS. It's about how to do things properly and how to work with others.

Each day will be filled with little dramas. You may be thanked, laughed at, moved to tears, congratulated and told off all in one morning! Sometimes you will feel like a hamster running around a wheel, but always remember that you are playing a small part in running this extraordinary organisation. Everything you do, however big or small, will have some impact on someone's life.

Controlled bleeping.

Dr A:"Where is Nurse X?"

Nurse in charge: "She's on break."

Dr A: "Forgive me for even mentioning her name!"

Nurse in charge: "Just this time, okay?"

Nurse X: "Where is Dr A?"

Nurse in charge: "At lunch"

Nurse X: "Fine, I'll bleep him"

Why does this happen to us and not to them? Because, nurses work smart. They talk to each other at handover, plan out their tasks and decide who is going to first break, second break etc. And during that time, they cannot be interrupted.

Yet over and over again I see doctors being bleeped, for miniscule things. I watch them get up to answer calls during lunch time and even during bleep-free teaching. Yet, the only thing that cannot wait is an acute emergency eg: a cardiac arrest/sepsis.

Suggestion

Now you know how to plan your day, tell the nurse in charge what you will be doing and where you will be. It's also a good idea to tell the Consultant's secretary or ward clerk too if you can. Tell them to batch up all the tasks for you while you will be on the ward. If you have teaching at lunch time, practise uttering this statement:

"At twelve thirty I will be attending bleep-free teaching. I will be off site for an hour. So, unless you fancy hearing the voice of the woman from postgrad, who is holding all the bleeps, don't call me."

Or

"Dear Sister, I am going for something to eat. I will be back in half an hour. I'm happy to do any jobs waiting when I come back and I'm happy for you to bleep me if it is a dire emergency. Now repeat after me *DIRE*!"

AS: Creating a "job book" can really help the nurses know where to write any non-urgent tasks and this way they don't have to chase you around. It only works if you keep checking it though!

Mindful working

Try and remember what it's like to be on the other side as a patient and what it's like for the other people you are working with. I will touch on some common issues encountered on a daily basis.

Complaints

Unless you are having a baby, a new kidney or a facelift, coming to hospital is a low point in someone's life. Stress is high. Little things really push people's buttons. And it's usually that stuff they complain about.

At junior level, you don't see the impact. By the time you've written their discharge summary, the patient is well and truly out of your head, but for many of them the suffering is ongoing.

Also, a Consultant and senior nurse may have to spend three hours each, going through a patient's notes answering a complaint, then attend a two-hour panel meeting. If it's serious, then the problem escalates to more meetings. A stack of complaints can be costly and really impact service delivery.

Look for the warning signs. A history of previous complaints. A patient who has had a nasty experience in the past. Pushy relatives. Someone with a carefully prepared list of questions or someone who seems unhappy with everything you say and do.

Answer the darn phone

This is actually something people complain about! I see juniors sitting by a ringing phone, deliberately ignoring it. Why? Because it's not their job to answer it.

But telling an anxious relative that their loved one is sitting up in bed eating breakfast takes ten seconds, and could really make someone's day. Telling endoscopy that the patient is ready takes five seconds. Imagine how much more quickly inpatient endoscopies could be done if staff didn't have to waste so much time hunting people down?

I would make it a point to answer three phone calls when you are by the phone. Not every phone call, just three. You will still make a difference.

Be mindful about how you act

Dr S "I didn't think twice about my short skirts and low-cut tops until I had to clerk a patient having a mastectomy. I realised that I was flaunting my femininity in front of someone who was just about to lose theirs. And she was my age."

Dr C "This is a fabulous teaching case, massive mitral valve vegetations, with a cracking murmur!"

How would you feel if Dr C and her pals are stood talking in front of YOU, while you're filling up with fluid and hoping that you won't stroke out? Not so fabulous eh?

AS: As someone who has a loud voice, and likes to talk, I always have to remind myself that the world is a small place. Talking through cases is good for learning and decompressing, but check if other people can hear you (e.g. in the canteen) and also take care with the kind of language you are using.

A member of the public made a complaint to my medical school when she overheard some medical students discussing patients' cases on the bus in town.

Who are you?

True story. The other day a young blond guy barged into an orthopaedic theatre and asked the surgeon if he could step in and perform the hip replacement. Despite the dangling ID badge, the surgeon had never seen the young blond guy in all of his life and the young blond guy had never met the patient, nor the surgeon.

For all the surgeon knew, the young blond guy could have been Leonardo Di Caprio in *'Catch Me if you Can'*. A movie about a fraudster who pretends to be among other things, a doctor.

The patient had seen this particular surgeon in his clinic twice in the past year. The surgeon had examined his hip, looked at the X Rays, counselled the patient and his family about the risks and benefits of the procedure. He had earned the patient's trust. Hence, the patient had given him his consent to perform the operation.

And what had this blond guy done? Turned up on the day wearing an ID badge, claiming that he needed his log book filled in.

Now can you understand why the surgeon got angry?

Suggestion

Please be respectful of the patient. If you wish to carry out an elective operation on someone, look at the X-rays, read up the clinical notes, see the patient first and contact the surgeon well in advance. It is a privilege that you earn, not a right.

Obviously, things work differently in an emergency. At the very least, introduce yourself to the surgical team if you are going to assist.

Mindful clerking

When you go on an overseas trip, you have to check in first, having typed in your name, address and passport number correctly. You have to have the right visas and travel documents. If you haven't done things properly, you won't be allowed through. End of story.

So how is it that in our organisation, people are allowed to enter the doors with flimsy, illegible scraps of paper, missing vital pieces of information, and sometimes without even a name on them, when they are about to make the most difficult journey in their life? And to top it all off, it's a legal document! One day when we have a fully electronic system, things might change.

The golden rules of mindful clerking

1. Patient's name and identification on each page.

2. Your name, grade and GMC number (get a stamp made and sign under it)

3. The date and time of your assessment

4. As much information as you can possibly fit in

The more information you put into your clerking, the more you, your hospital, your patient and all the other people looking after them will get out of it, (yes, even in Orthopaedics).

Most places now have a standardised admission pro-forma. But please put in as much detail as you can.

Look at old discharge summaries and clinic letters to help you. And think of it as a passport application form. If it is not filled in properly, nobody gets anywhere.

Exercise: Look at the table below.

Now imagine patient A and patient B coming into hospital. Someone does a hasty clerking and scribbles down the same shopping list of conditions for each of them, even though it's different.

Shopping list style past history	past history of Patient A	past history of Patient B
IHD	MI 20 years ago, nil angina since, Effort tolerance 3 MILES	MI 3 months ago

PCI Rt coronary artery

Dual antiplatelets until: |
| DIABETES | Controlled with diet

Hba1c 50 mmol/mol | Type 1 diabetes, poor control

Peripheral neuropathy |
| COPD | prn Inhalers, ET 3 miles not smoked 20 years | Current smoker

Uses home Nebulisers

Effort Tolerance 20 yards |
| CKD | EGFR 64 | CKD stage 4 EGFR 29

Planned fistula |
| HERNIA REPAIR | Left inguinal hernia 10 years ago, uncomplicated mesh repair | Obstructed left inguinal hernia

10 years ago, partial resection small bowel |

Now what would happen if each of them

- fractured their neck of femur or

- had a GI bleed on the ward or

- became acutely confused or

- had a respiratory arrest and were being considered for intensive care

Can you see what a difference those extra few sentences of description can make?

- To a surgeon deciding to operate

- To the Endoscopist

- To the junior doctor coming into review the patient (which might be you)

- To a person's life

AS: How often do you spend a dedicated 30 to 45 minutes on one patient during a hospital admission? Usually only when clerking. And it doesn't matter whether it's Orthopaedics or Surgical either. Get it right the first time. Catch a snapshot of the person, not just their list of co-morbidities. As someone who has to go to arrest calls, I can understand how vital the social history is and often it isn't even filled in!

You don't want to take forever, because the real emergency may be sitting quietly in a corner having a silent MI. But clerking is a golden opportunity to get crucial information. It also gets you talking to people and learning all about them. That was one of the reasons you went into medicine, right?

But there are ten waiting and they are going to breach!

Please remember that you are responsible for the patient you are currently seeing and the patients you have seen. Patients will continue pouring in and in busy periods, there will be nurses and Bed managers breathing down your neck, saying things like: "If you see Mr X quickly then he can go up to a ward."

Trap! Don't fall for it! When you do things quickly, you are more likely to make mistakes. And those nurses or Bed managers won't be there to hold your hand at the disciplinary hearing if you ever require one.

Beware of drug charts and allergies. Make sure that you've written insulin doses and times correctly (shorting acting and pre-mixed insulin should be given with meals and NEVER before bed).

AS: When it's super busy, you have to adapt. I adapt by becoming very focussed. When clerking, I minimise the time spent looking at old clinic letters, get the facts and move on. I will make sure I have done everything (X-ray forms, drug charts) before moving on to another patient and I keep a list of jobs I need to go back to.

If there is only 15 minutes before the end of my shift, then I see if I can help someone else by writing a drug chart for them or scribing for them while they take a history. This can help speed things up.

Doing the job versus getting the job done

Surgeon: "So where is the scan?"

Junior doctor: "I sent the request form down"

Surgeon: "I DIDN'T ASK IF YOU HAD SENT THE REQUEST FORM DOWN, I ASKED FOR THE SCAN!"

You've done your bit, you've handed in a request form to Radiology, but the scan hasn't been done. The surgeon needs the scan before operating, the patient has been starved, the anaesthetist, theatre space and ITU bed have been booked. So, without the scan the whole system is about to collapse and you are about to get shouted at.

Stop! Rewind! To try and prevent this scenario, you should understand that things do not happen seamlessly in the NHS. You will often have to go the extra mile to get a job done and, in the process, you will learn how to badger, annoy and beg.

In the case of urgent X-rays and scans, you may need to go down to the Radiology department and discuss the case with the Radiologist face to face, so they can prioritise your patient. Obviously, you cannot do this for everyone, but certainly for the acutely ill patients and the ones going to theatre.

WARNING! Some Radiologists bite.

They are less likely to do so if you know the full clinical details and can clearly state the reasons for your visit. If they do bite, try not to take it personally. They are probably just overstretched and fed up. If they refuse to prioritise your scan, ask them nicely to explain why, document it and inform your Consultant. There is usually a very good reason.

Similarly, Biochemistry and Haematology labs process thousands of samples per day, but if you contact them directly and explain to them the 'story' behind the super urgent request, then the patient is no longer a 'number' in a queue. For example, you could call and tell them "Can you run this blood sample quickly please? This lady is 32 weeks pregnant with twins and bleeding."

These folks don't have quite the same reputation as Radiologists though and are generally much easier to deal with. Sometimes, they might even be grateful for human contact.

Mindful discharging

When I was a junior doctor sending someone home, I would imagine a silver-haired GP sitting eagerly on a black swivel chair, arms open wide, ready to receive my patient, like a rugby player waiting for a pass. And of course, they were just dying to read every word of my discharge summary and carry out each instruction with a smile.

I was clueless.

Many practices are staffed by locums, who would not know the patient from Adam, and sometimes the discharge summaries are read by clerical staff and practice nurses. Or not at all.

GPs need to know the diagnosis, investigations, medications and follow up plan. And a self-caring patient / relative / carer needs to know the same. And as in the previous section, you will have to figure out how the jobs are actually going to get done after discharge.

An instruction like "We'll ask the GP to repeat bloods in three days and follow up in a week",is pointless if the practice nurse can't do the blood test until five days and the earliest doctor's appointment is in three weeks.

AS: Sometimes the advice can be overwhelming, it needs to be written out and handed to the patient with the discharge summary eg: when to have bloods, when to see the GP etc

Mindful surgical discharging

If you are discharging someone after an operation, lay out clear instructions as to the timing of suture removal, duration of antibiotic therapy, and follow up. Find out exactly when the patient needs to be reviewed and where and how this will happen. Also, please find out if there are any additional instructions which are **specific** to the procedure they have had, such as duration of anti-platelet therapy. If you are not sure, look it up or ask. For example, if the person has had a total thyroidectomy, what specific drugs do they need? The answer is definitely Thyroxine and possibly also calcium and Vitamin D analogues.

Mindful clinic letter writing

Secretary A: "In future, can you make sure Doctor X only sees two patients per clinic, because I've just spent forty-five minutes typing one of his letters!"

Secretary B: "Many doctors actually cough while dictating, without bothering to turn the machine off. Don't they realise that we're wearing headphones when we type, and that it blasts our eardrums!"

When you are dictating a clinic letter, think of the person typing it and the person reading it. Except in special situations such as a detailed case review, post mortem, neurology or psychiatric consultation, the clinic letter should be brief.

Suggested format: "Wham, bam thank you Mam!"

Diagnosis

Treatment

Brief clinical note including test results

Follow up/future plan.

"But that's my European day."

So, there's a difficult operation happening, something that you rarely get the chance to see or assist with. Or there are two people awaiting lumbar punctures and you need to practise. It's unfortunate that these things clash with your European working time directive day off. (This day may have to be renamed after Brexit). It's your loss if you don't come in.

AS: It is hard, but I would suggest using your private study leave allowance for that kind of thing. It will be bleep free then. I've also moved my EWTD day over to when it was more convenient and when there were more team members around to cover.

Learning when to zone out and when to listen

Medics are competitive by nature. Many of us have been driven along by pushy parents and expectant teachers. We've soared through our classes with straight As, collected various prizes and graduated from medical school with flying colours.

But the real world works differently. Suddenly you may find yourself falling behind in the 'race' to get ahead. Or, after being complimented and congratulated all your life, people start questioning your judgment and telling you what to do.

People who haven't been spent years at medical school, or won prizes.

One of the greatest skills you will ever acquire, is knowing when to zone out and not listen, and when to 'be humble' and listen.

It gets easier as you get older, I promise.

When not to listen

"Thirty-five and still not married! When are you going to have children?"

"I can't believe you haven't applied for a Consultant job!"

"How many times have you sat the Part 1 now? Do you intend to keep going with it?"

"You've only got one publication so far?"

Right now, you might be thirty-five and living with your tortoise. Next year, you may meet someone and become an awesome step-parent. You may not be interested in a Consultant job right away because you want to join The American Red Cross for a year.

Do you think the patients in your future speciality will ever want to know how many times you sat the Part 1? You may choose to keep going until you pass. Equally you may decide that after three attempts you will pursue option B, whatever that is.

Every life is unique. Each trajectory you create is your own. Just by working as a doctor you are making an important contribution to society.

So, ignore those voices and zone out.

AS: Loved ones might be genuinely concerned about you. Sometimes they just forget that they are not you! But others who ask you about the number of papers you've published or number of times you've sat an exam may simply be trying to psych you out or just trying to reassure themselves.

When to listen

Podiatrist: "I'm rather concerned that his foot is getting worse despite the fact that he's already on antibiotics. Don't you think he needs admission?"

Junior Doctor: "He's not systemically unwell, so I'm discharging him."

Nurse: "I am worried about her. Something about her colour. Should we re-check an Hb?"

Junior Doctor: "I've already checked it. It's 95."

Once upon a time a nurse was looked upon as a doctor's obedient side-kick. Thankfully the nursing profession has advanced exponentially. Nurse practitioners and specialist nurses have a wealth of knowledge and experience. You will also meet other allied health professionals like podiatrists and physiotherapists who have years of experience with patients.

As a junior doctor, you may be tempted to ignore words of advice from such people. Sometimes it's professional pride. Sometimes you are just too busy.

But these are precisely the voices you need to listen to. They have been in the game far longer than you have.

p.s.Both scenarios occurred during the time of writing. The first patient ended up in ITU in another hospital, with sepsis. The second patient did have a haemoglobin of 95 in the morning, but later in the day it had dropped to 62.

TO WRAP UP

We hope this little book will be a useful companion for you and that after reading it you will:

- take care of your physical and mental health

- be time aware, with a rough idea of how to plan out your day and week

- make a conscious effort to fill *all* your boxes

- do some proper investigating into career pathways (and NOT just ask one Obstetrics Registrar why he chose his job, believe him when he tells you "it's easy", then curse and blame him five years later)

- work smarter

And most of all, we hope that after 'surviving' your junior doctor years, you will not only become a successful doctor, but a successful person who is a doctor. One who lives well and works well. Alongside others. For others. And of course, for YOU.

Sincerely,
Dr Moushmi Biswas and Dr Anna Scholz

ABOUT THE AUTHORS

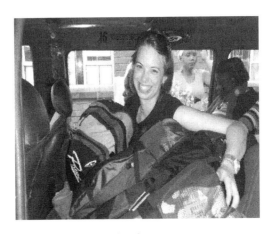

AS in her happy space

Anna Scholz is a specialty trainee in Endocrinology and Diabetes. She did her undergraduate degree in dreamy Oxford, and later discovered beautiful Wales. Currently, she has given into her geeky side and is undertaking a part-time MD about the thyroid and brain. To relax, she loves to scuba dive in far flung places, play guitar and catch up with friends and eat yummy food. To practise what she preaches to her patients, and counteract her love of food, she has recently started jogging. Whilst plodding round the park, she hopes to learn Spanish so she can run a half marathon before going diving in South America. Oh, and she also wants to achieve Consultant-hood before she's forty.

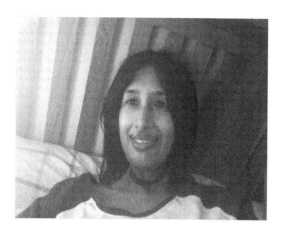

MB Favourite place. Favourite clothing.

Moushmi Biswas is a Consultant Physician in Diabetes, Endocrinology and Internal Medicine. She was born in West Brom and did her early schooling in the Midlands. Her family then moved to Australia. After a stint in the outback, she studied Medicine in Sydney and came back to the UK. She got her MRCP in 1998 and CCT in2005.

In case you were asking, she did try to return to Oz, but was not happy to re-sit exams and re-train. So, she took up a Consultant post at the Royal Gwent and then decided to do an MD (the wrong way round), on Testosterone and Diabetes, eventually becoming the oldest person to graduate.

She lives in Cardiff with her partner, her son and their naughty little dog. Like Anna S, she loves eating yummy food with her mates, but then has to go carb free.

Her first novel entitled '*Maple and Spice*', a transcontinental romp, a bit like '*Bridget Jones*' meets '*the Exotic Marigold Hotel*', was published in 2018.

Also by this Author

"Maple and Spice",
published 2018 Matador Books.

Monisha Bastikar is twenty-seven years old and has just finished medical school in Vermont. She has three shining goals: to become a wife, a mother and a board-certified Physician. But time is running out, the men in her community are taken and residency at the prestigious St Anthony's is just around the corner.

Monisha's over-ambitious mother Leela tells her all is not lost, for in India there are millions of men. Monisha opts for an arranged marriage, leaving her best friend Tina completely bewildered. Mrs Bastikar and her feisty younger sister Aunt Romila trawl through the Mumbai Matrimonials and shortlist Shailesh Kulkarni, a dashing surgeon, with glittering career prospects. On paper he appears to be the perfect match and Monisha can't believe her luck.

But all is not what it seems and Monisha is faced with some difficult choices. Should she break with cultural traditions and find love the American way, or should she compromise and keep her family happy?

The search for love takes Monisha on an eventful journey tinged with heartbreak and loss, from Vermont to Mumbai and back again. Eventually she abandons all hope and throws herself into her career. But will she sit back and wait for a prince to rescue her or will she find the courage to rescue herself?

Maple and Spice is a light-hearted, tragi-comic romp through love and relationships in the twenty-first, century. It also explores the themes of cultural identity, female empowerment and self-fulfilment.

Available as an e-book on Amazon Kindle and on Google Play

https://www.troubador.co.uk/bookshop/romance/maple-and-spice/

'A touching book with beautiful characters that the author made you feel were true to life, vivid and honest. The storyline captured your mind and transports you to a different country and way of life where ancient customs and rituals play a huge part in modern life. Sad and poignant at times but with some fantastic life lessons and an insight into a world of hope and high expectations. A must read from a fabulous new author.'

Gayle Goldstein, Net Galley

'...A cross culture roller coaster ride of happiness and dis-appointment. The author's writing style allowed you to be sympathetic to the central character and her choices because that's how life can be. There are some serious social issues which the author explores and at the same

time it had elements of a Nick Hornby novel with a Bollywood bent. A stellar effort for a first novel.'

John Rooney

Printed in Great Britain
by Amazon